How to Become a Personal Trainer

The Ultimate Guide to Establishing a Successful Personal Training Career

by **K.B. Bryson**

Table of Contents

Introduction..... 1

Chapter 1: Education and Certification Requirements
....7

Chapter 2: The Foundation of a Successful Personal
Trainer 11

Chapter 3: Qualities of Great Trainers While
Training...19

Chapter 4: Gym Employment Vs. Self-Employment
....29

Chapter 5: Tips for Marketing Your Business 33

Conclusion 37

Introduction

A personal training career is characterized by a single word – *passion*. Have you had a burning passion for fitness throughout your life? Do you possess that desire to coax others toward healthier living, to cajole them towards a more balanced outlook and a greater sense of physical achievement? If you were the kid who loved trying out the latest piece of equipment on the playground or in gym class, or even if you discovered the joys of physical fitness at some later point in your life and unearthed a deep-seated wish to spread that joy – this is the perfect career for you!

However, a personal fitness trainer isn't just a drill sergeant; he or she is also a client's guide, companion, supporter, and therapist. A fitness trainer isn't a bully, and certainly isn't some old monk driving young initiates through the gauntlets of Hell in an effort to pass on some vague esoteric wisdom. Those initiates did not have the opportunity to leave their master behind without resigning their very identity. But your clients *do,* and some will take that opportunity at the first possible instance, which basically spells the doom of your career. A successful personal fitness trainer is more like Yoda – a fearsome warrior, a support figure, and an unparalleled scholar of the trade, all rolled into one.

So, what differentiates a successful and capable trainer from one who enters the field full of enthusiasm with guns blazing, but gets run off the board in no time? What aspects of business, as well as unorthodox mental perspectives must a physical trainer understand to make the most of themselves and their abilities in the professional world?

These are precisely the questions that I'm going to address in this guide, so that between *your* passion and knowledge and *my* understanding of the business world – we can set you up to become a legendary trainer in no time. Are you ready to unlock the secrets of great personal fitness experts? Are you ready to separate yourself from the glorified jocks, and get on your way to becoming a fitness guru? If so, let's get started!

Chapter 1: Education and Certification Requirements

For some strange reason, many newcomers aspiring to become fitness trainers believe that being buff, roaming around in tight polo t-shirts, gym pants and colorful sneakers, and spending inordinate amounts of time flexing muscles in the gym is all that it takes to be a successful fitness trainer. However, this could not be further from the truth.

As befits a field which deals with the health and welfare of the human body, the profession of fitness training is heavily regulated, and requires several necessary certifications before you can pursue it as a career. This shouldn't come as a surprise to you. A good fitness trainer needs to know the human body and its normative bio-mechanical functions just as well as a doctor, if not more in some cases. Great trainers are expected not only to know each muscle group in the human body and ways to develop them efficiently, but also their points of attachment and the natural paths and angles along which each muscle group should contract and expand during normative movement. They're also expected to be familiar with various body types and shapes, and the associated metabolic activity which goes hand-in-hand with each, as well as the best training methods which tend to work well for those sets of parameters.

Nothing is more harmful than half-truths, and fitness trainers who half-ass their knowledge won't just be metaphorically harming their clients. They could be putting them at risk for serious injuries in a very literal sense.

Keeping this in mind, once you have a high school diploma, you should look at certification courses relevant to the fitness world that are recognized by the NCCA (National Commission for Certifying Agencies). Some of the most widely popular recognized organizations tending to certification needs are the American Council on Exercise, Aerobics & Fitness Association of America, National Federation of Professional Trainers, the AFPA (American Fitness Professionals and Associates) and the National Academy of Sports and Medicine. Keep in mind that such certifying bodies usually have their own educational requirements and membership criteria.

In keeping with the intense competitive atmosphere of the business world in modern times, newcomers to the fitness industry who hold recognized graduate degrees pertaining to Exercise Physiology & Sciences, Sports Medicine, Diet & Nutrition and other such relevant course certifications would have an edge over others during the search for employment opportunities. So, as soon as you complete your degree, check out the minimum requirements for different certification bodies and start grinding away at their exams. You'll thank yourself for doing so later – and so will your pocketbook.

Also, apart from your graduate degree and any post-graduate or accompanying diplomas which you may choose to seek out for before you start working, you also need to be certified in the use of Automated External Defibrillators (AED) and Cardiopulmonary Resuscitation (CPR) techniques, since you may come across clients with medical conditions who suffer an emergency during a training session. Being ready to assist in this type of event is a must.

These form the base of your educational and certification requirements, after which you can search for employment in gyms or open a personal training business of your own. However, by no means is this the end of your learning – enhancing your foundation of knowledge will continue for as long as you wish to remain at the top of your field. We'll discuss more about that later on.

Chapter 2: The Foundation of a Successful Personal Trainer

There are a handful of physical, mental, and emotional attributes which form the foundation of a great personal trainer. These are the bedrock upon which their successful career is established.

[1] A Great Fitness Trainer Is Always in Shape. Period

This point is rather obvious, yet important nonetheless. As a fitness trainer, you have to lead by example. Now, this doesn't mean that you have to look like a Rock Troll from Mars. But your physique has to effectively display the aesthetics of fitness. Keep in mind that the training you'll have to go through will push your body into realms of shape beyond that of a normal person, but your own physical fitness is the biggest testimonial to your capabilities as a trainer. If you start slipping and get soft, you *will* lose out on present and prospective future clients. And understandably so! How comfortable would you feel if your dentist had crooked, yellow teeth? Exactly.

[2] A Great Fitness Trainer Is Always Up to Date

The most successful trainers have reached their levels of professional achievement primarily because they're passionate about what they do. It's not just a job to them. Rather, it is something they're *genuinely* interested in pursuing. This reflects in their never-ending urge to absorb any new piece of information about their professional art – be it medical or scientific journals, professional feedback on new and upcoming technologies or equipment, or even new exercise techniques and routines. They are always on the lookout to push their understanding of their field further, and to polish their craft at every given opportunity.

That's why great trainers not only spend time developing their bodies, but also their minds. They voraciously devour any books, magazines, journals and articles relevant to their fields that they can lay their hands on in their free time. If this isn't a habit that you can get on board with, you might as well switch to another field right now. Or get a name tag that says "Mediocre."

Not only are the best trainers always updated, but they sign up for new courses, certifications, seminars, and workshops as often as they can. Instead of viewing such activities as unnecessary expenses, the best trainers always think of such avenues as investments into maintaining a professionally relevant set of skills.

[3] While Competitive Pricing Is Important, Great Trainers Charge Based on Their Worth

Since this is a one-on-one job that requires hands-on work with your clients, it's always important to maintain a suitably accurate understanding of the value of skills that you bring to the table.

Although newer trainers are always worried about the prices of their competition, the most successful trainers understand that people don't mind paying a bit extra if they feel they're getting their money's worth. With this in mind, you should still always know your competitor's offers and pricing.

Do your background research on your competitors in the area. Ask to meet up with them personally; or if they're unwilling, simply have a friend call them up as a potential client and get a feel for the services they provide and their value for the fee that they charge.

If you feel that you may not have as much to offer yet, you can definitely price yourself a little lower than the market average to ensure larger incentives for your clients. However, if you feel you have more to offer, then don't hesitate to mark up your fee 10 to 15% higher than the competition. Since you're only charging for what you can practically deliver, you'll be able to guarantee customer satisfaction without any problems.

[4] Great Trainers Are Always in Business Mode

The most successful trainers understand that they're in a people-oriented profession, and so having a business plan in mind is always crucial. They don't shirk away from treating their profession like a business. They also aren't satisfied with simply following the business plans of their gym or other such place of employment, and are constantly on the look-out for opportunities which may help them take their profession into their own hands, rather than relying on fitness organizations that end up taking a huge chunk of their money anyway.

Even though you may be in gym attire, visualize yourself in a slick business suit instead. You're not some high-school jock constantly hitting the gym. You're actually a businessperson looking for ways to establish yourself on your own two feet. If you don't develop your entrepreneurial skills, or try to formulate your own business model, you'll always be stuck at a mediocre level.

[5] Great Trainers Make Their Clients Feel Important

To make this point clear, this does *not* mean that you make a client feel important simply by pandering to them. Instead, great trainers make their clients feel as though they're always at the forefront of their trainers' minds.

The simplest way to do this is to keep in touch with your client outside training. However, this isn't so that you can send them inane forwards and silly jokes. Whenever you come across some interesting reading material about fitness, and think a particular client could benefit from it, email it to them. You can also send them nutritional charts or dietary articles from which you believe they would benefit.

Also, keep in mind any personal details or events in their lives which may be coming up, and follow up on them – like a vacation, upcoming nuptials, etc. And during the next training session, ask specific questions like "Hey, how was your trip to Panama with your wife and daughter?"

15

If they've had a particularly great training session, congratulate them and put up a post commending them for their hard work on their Facebook wall. Not only will that make them happier to have received your approval, but it also will market your services to anyone who can see the post on their wall.

If you're ever bending rules for a client because they're unwell, or helping them out by waiving any deduction from a last-minute no-show because they're sick, make sure they know you're doing them a favor. Tell them, "My policy is normally X, but for you I'll do Y, but just this once."

[6] Great Trainers Bite Off Only as Much as They Can Chew

This is particularly true in case you're self employed. The best trainers understand the need to not face burnout caused by over-booked schedules or troublesome clients. Only promise what you can deliver. If you have the slightest hesitation about delivering in the promised timeframe, then refrain from making a commitment. Also, if you're taking on clients who just don't mesh well with you, either transfer them to another colleague (suggesting another trainer would be a better fit) or simply let the client go altogether. You'll do your best work when

16

you're training clients who energize you rather than drain you. It's best for everyone involved – trust me.

When you're working on your own, you also need to regulate and fix the maximum number of hours you're able to work for each day, or else the exhaustion will surely wear you down. And if that happens, your clients will pick up on it, and you'll eventually lose business because of it.

Chapter 3: Qualities of Great Trainers While Training

[1] Great Fitness Trainers Check Their Ego at the Door

As I mentioned before, fitness trainers aren't bullies — they're Yodas. The best fitness trainers understand that clients place their well-being in a trainer's hands in the trust that they'll be guided towards what's best for them. This means that if a client isn't agreeing to follow your every suggestion and pointer, it's because you haven't convinced them enough so far to make them follow you without question.

At no point should your ego be a factor in any interaction you have with a client. If your client doesn't seem to follow your pointers, find alternate methods of getting through to them instead of escalating the situation or giving up on them.

[2] A Great Fitness Trainer Is Adaptable

One of the largest mistakes that many trainers make is they keep pushing techniques and methods that worked for them onto their clients. This is a particularly disastrous mistake to make.

Even if Routine A worked for you and every other client you've worked with, it might not work for your very next one. The best fitness trainers don't rely on two or three set routines to choose from when they deal with clients. Instead, they understand the objective of every exercise component in a routine, and retain knowledge about a sufficiently diverse array of techniques so as to be able to come up with a tailored fitness routine for each and every one of their clients.

Example: If you're well-versed in techniques and equipment "A" to "Z", maybe a combination of "A", "C", "H", and a diet 'I' may work best for a client, while "B", "C", "F", "S" and diet "Q" might work better for another.

This is precisely why the most successful trainers are always up to date on any new tools, techniques, and research which may be revealed through professional journals with relevance to the fitness industry. Doing so also requires you to check your ego, admit to yourself when you've made a mistake regarding the needs of a client, and switch over to better-suited methods as soon as you possibly can if such situations should arise.

[3] A Great Fitness Trainer Knows the Client's Goals

Another thing that's overlooked by many trainers is the simple act of knowing the client's goals. This doesn't just mean how much weight they'd like to lose, or how buff they want to appear, but most importantly...by when?

Dissatisfaction from a client usually occurs when they feel their goals aren't being met. But the simple truth is that many clients have unrealistic goals. Too much time spent watching training montages in movies makes people think they can get ripped in a month, and they bring those same expectations to their training sessions. At this point, no matter how good you may be, or however effectively you may be doing your job, you will not be able to satisfy your client's desires. Eventually, the client will simply blame you for not being able to meet their goals and discontinue your services. Be prepared for this.

You can avoid this though by talking to your client about their goals on the very first day. The best trainers use this to get a feel of their client's motivations as well, correct them in order to make goals more realistic, as well as create a step by step plan detailing how those goals can be practically achieved.

21

Once you've done this, you've essentially broken down the journey into bite-sized steps for the client, and given them milestones to look forward to which would motivate them during hard training sessions. You've also assured that you're promising exactly what you can deliver to your client, which will increase your credibility and perceived performance greatly.

[4] A Great Fitness Trainer Quantifies Everything

The best trainers understand that nothing incentivizes a person more strongly than an understanding of how far they've come since day one. With this in mind, when you take on a new client, get as much 'before' data as you possibly can – photos, measurements, etc.

From that point on, keep updating that data regularly to show your client every improvement they've made. A lot of people aren't naturally oriented to taking fitness seriously, and when such people come to you as clients it becomes all the more important to keep giving them a sense of accomplishment whenever possible. Imagine a client who weighs herself daily, constantly discouraged because she hasn't lost a pound. Think of how great she'll feel when you point out (and can prove) that her waist shrunk by four inches!

[5] A Great Fitness Trainer Is Supportive

While it may sometimes become important to be your client's drill-sergeant, the necessity of that situation ever arising also shows that adequate communication or trust with the client may still be lacking. Regardless, if you're ever hard on your clients, it's also just as important to be a soft supporter too.

Whenever your client does something well, or makes an extra effort, or gets something right – make a big deal about it. Show your support by showing your clients that you do keep your utmost attention on them, and are ready to compliment their achievements without reserve.

This fosters a deeper bond between client and trainer, and urges a client to work harder for you, since they'll value your opinion and approval on fitness matters.

[6] A Great Trainer Generalizes *and* Specializes

A great trainer understands that people would rather train under a multi-talented professional than search for new ones all the time to suit their different needs. Many people advise that specialization is key in creating a successful business today. However, that is far from the truth. As I mentioned earlier, great trainers need to be adaptable. To fulfill that need, you must have a thorough understanding and success with plenty of diverse exercises and equipment so that you can create tailored fitness routines for each individual client.

Having said that, you've got to continue developing your skills sets, as well as absorb as much knowledge about different fitness-related matters as possible. With this in mind, it's necessary to be somewhat generalized about what you can offer to your clients while constantly pursuing specializations on your own time.

This is particularly vital in your first 5 to 10 years as a personal fitness trainer. Many great trainers, after they start working, choose at least one certification every year and keep working on it on their own time until they can add that to their list of skills by the end of the year. This way, every year will see your skill sets on the rise, and increase the amount of value for money you bring to the table, which will also enable you to increase your fees. The ultimate goal isn't just to be the trainer that people *only* approach for a specific goal, i.e. becoming the trainer they approach *only* when they need to work out on the Kettle bell. Your objective should be to become the person everyone approaches in the hopes that their desired preferences may be one of the paths which you're quite knowledgeable about and experienced in.

Thus, generalize when coming up with your client's fitness routine, but keep specializing yourself every year.

[7] Great Trainers Strive to Make Themselves Redundant

Now, this point is rather counter-intuitive, and many trainers tend to trip up here. However, you need to remember that your primary job is to foster a healthy outlook in your client's physical activities. You won't always be there to keep an eye on whether or not they're sticking to the program, and your clients are a reflection of your skills as a trainer – this is especially true when they may be suggesting you as a trainer to others. A lot of trainers, fearing the redundancy and losing their clientele as a result, hold back their advice and instruction, and don't impart a lot of wisdom that would otherwise allow their client to flourish.

The problem with that is many such clients are quite slow at getting to their goals in such cases, and thus blame the trainer, lose motivation, and quit. Instead of turning your client into a money-minting puppet, foster the importance and need for fitness that burns inside you in your clients as well. If they get healthier and fitter on their own time by following advice given to them by you, they'll be giving you the credit nonetheless. Not only that, but the positive associations which would then be linked in their minds with being under your tutelage would probably guarantee return and continued patronage because they'd automatically associate being healthier with working out under you.

[8] The Best Trainers Are Human. Not Muscle-Bound Robots

The best trainers understand that, while fear has traditionally been a good tool to spur clients on in the past, the best way to get someone to push themselves beyond their usual physical limits is to do it for someone they like and respect and with whom they have fun. Trainers who can laugh, joke, and socialize with their clients do far better in terms of results and client loyalty than others. Also, trainers should not be above leading by example and hitting the weights with their client once in a while.

For example, if a client is unable to push himself far enough to meet his target for abdomen crunches over a few days, join him in going through his exercises for the day while matching him set for set.

Your job is not to make the gym terrifying, but rather a fun place with which clients can foster a positive association.

Chapter 4: Gym Employment Vs. Self-Employment

There are various pros and cons attached to both paths. However, we will discuss both of them below, and it will be up to you to determine the course that works best for you.

Gym Employment – Gymnasiums offer credibility and experience, as well as an understanding of how the fitness business runs from the grassroots level.

Most clients prefer choosing personal trainers who have worked in well-known gyms at one point or the other. While this may not be entirely sensible to those of you contemplating starting off as self-employed, let me ask you this: would you prefer a doctor who did his internship and residency after finishing his studies, or one who came straight from his books and was immediately assigned to diagnosing you without any notable practical experience? Choosing to work for a gym will also stabilize your income, as well as provide a steady stream of clients to work with. Since you're a newcomer to the world of fitness, gyms also steady your position and prevent you from dropping yourself into a make-or-break situation.

On the other hand, gyms take away your chance to screen your customers, and take a rather large portion of your income regardless. They may also restrict your ability to try out your own tailor-made fitness routines on clients.

Self-Employed – Since you've already completed your graduation and certifications, there's no doubt that you're already set up to be able to start your own personal fitness training business. Whether you run the training out of your own space, or provide training sessions at your clients' homes, the path of the self-employed requires a lot more hard work, dedication, and business cunning.

However, it gives you full creative freedom with fitness routines – in keeping with updated knowledge – and also prevents large chunks of your money from being taken by the gym.

The self-employed path also gives you the capacity to develop your own marketing and advertising strategies, as well as develop a client base that's solely loyal to you for its fitness needs, rather than to a gym.

Chapter 5: Tips for Marketing Your Business

[1] Be Your Own Billboard

Whether you work in a gym or for yourself, always remember that you're the best advertising for yourself. Get polo t-shirts from your gym, or get some made with your own logo if you're self-employed. Wear them wherever you go. Remember that if you just start looking for clients by the time you desperately need their business, you're too late.

[2] Use Your Network

Everybody has a network of friends, relatives, and family through social media sites and other such means. However, the difference between mediocre and successful fitness instructors is the degree to which they've plumbed their network. Contact your friends and family and ask them to spread the word of your business to anyone who may require your services.

Offer referrals bonuses to people you know for every person they send your way.

[3] Identify Neighborhood Opinion Leaders

These people don't need to be at the top or the bottom of the social rung, but are usually in professions which allow them the distinct advantage of being able to drop a word here and there while interacting with a multitude of people every day.

These are usually people like coffee shop staff, real estate agents, barbers and hairdressers in salons, etc. Regardless of whether you work in a gym or are allowed to do so, you can offer them discounts or referral bonuses for every person they send your way. If your gym doesn't approve, simply promise them 5% or so from the joining fee of every client that they send over to you.

[4] Keep Providing Offers

Marketing requires that you keep coming up with interesting deals and discounts throughout the year. Maintain a list of every prospective customer who's approached you before, every past or present client, as well as every neighborhood opinion leader that you've approached in your attempt to drum up more business. Send them offers for one free session, or 20% off on three referrals, or a lesson at half price for their spouse and kids, etc. The more aggressive you are when marketing, the higher your chances are of staying in the forefront of their minds. Once you get them in, you can show them in person – through an unparalleled workout – how much they'll benefit from continuing to use your services.

Conclusion

While the world of personal fitness trainers is definitely an interesting one, it's also supremely competitive, and many people often switch over to another profession after the 3-year mark.

However, it's also extremely easy to understand as long as you remember the purpose of a personal fitness trainer. Don't ever be one of those people who think turning your nose up and getting 'annoyed with business stuff' should be an available option to you, since that would spell doom for your career from the outset.

Use every bit of your charisma and charm, (along with the network you've worked to amass) to push through and utilize the people in your network to market as efficiently as possible.

Above all, if you wish to be successful, three tips stand out from the rest:

1) Always keep yourself updated

2) Always remain flexible in training programs

3) Always make your client feel important

Also, do not overlook the fact that some certifications possess specific academic criteria which may need to be renewed or further worked upon every year for them to remain valid.

And one more thing… HAVE FUN! Always remember the reason that you became a personal fitness trainer in the first place, and make your workouts as fun as possible to get your clients healthier faster with less mental resistance. If done right, your career as a personal fitness trainer will ensure that *everyone* wins.

Last, thanks a lot for buying this book and taking the time to read it. I really hope that you found this guide informative, and I believe that if you follow my advice, you will certainly be successful as a personal trainer. If you found the book helpful, please be so kind as to leave a review on Amazon – I'd greatly appreciate it!

Made in United States
Troutdale, OR
10/03/2023

13375218R10027